CONTENTS

This book is presented as a collection of natural remedies and as an aid in understanding their use. It is not intended to replace or supersede professional consultation or treatment and no guarantee can be given as to the efficacy or appropriateness of a remedy in an individual case without professional advice.

INTRODUCTION

The purpose of this booklet is to inform and empower people so that they are able to understand depression better and know how to apply holistic remedies to relieve it.

Recent years have seen an explosion in the numbers of people who are experiencing symptoms of depression and requesting support in how to deal with it. According to the Mental Health Foundation, 1 in 6 people will be classified as depressed at some time in their life, although nearly everyone will experience some of the symptoms of depression at some point. This is reflected in the increasing use of prescribed medications despite there being considerable concern over their side effects.

Depression is most common in people aged 25-44 years although in the US, up to one and a half per cent of children between 2 and 4 years of age are given anti-depressants, including Prozac, and even more powerful drugs. The numbers of such prescriptions increased three times between 1991 and 1995 despite these drugs not being approved for children under the age of 6 years .

The cost to national health budgets is extreme. In the UK, some £100 million per year is spent on drugs to affect mood. This is 25 per cent of the national drug budget. The use of conventional medication, although perhaps necessary in some extreme states of mind, merely deals with the symptoms – the effect – rather than the cause.

HOLISTIC MEDICINE

Despite the impact, it is important to state that depression is not an illness and certainly not a disease. It is an emotion and one that we all experience from time to time. It is only when it becomes more severe and interferes with our functioning, that it may be labelled as a 'problem'. There are, however, many approaches that are on offer to ease depression and holistic medicine is a safe and effective choice.

In holistic medicine, we seek to nurture, balance and nourish the whole person. Any symptom – be it physical or psychological – is eased through considering the total picture of who the person is and what they need. There are two things that we, as humans, need for healing to take place: time and attention. Time we know about and even have sayings such as, 'Time is a great healer'. However, by itself this is not enough. We also need attention. We need to give ourselves and others that quality of attention, caring and of nurturing that enables us to truly find peace and tranquility.

Holistic medicine has always sought to see symptoms within the context of an integrated whole, and it is lifestyle changes that will be just as important as anything medicinal when improving depression. Self-help measures such as relaxation, yoga, tai chi or many other contemplative methods can be an essential part of any program seeking to relieve depression.

COMMON FACTORS IN DEPRESSION

When someone is diagnosed with depression, it is considered that some of the following are present:
· Guilt and low self-esteem
· Lack of interest in social activities and relationships
· Pessimistic outlook
· Thoughts or feelings of suicide
· Disturbed sleep which may include early morning wakening
· Poor memory, poor concentration
· Persistent feelings of sadness, low mood
· Physical symptoms which include tiredness, fatigue, appetite changes, headaches, digestive disorders, aches and pains

Not all people with depression will have all these symptoms as we are all different in our personalities and our reactions to events. It is helpful to consider that depression has different qualities and expressions.

ANTIDEPRESSANT USE

Conventionally, antidepressants are frequently used to treat depression and there were 8.5 million prescriptions for antidepressants in the UK in 1989 rising to 23.4 million in 1998. Their use is controversial particularly in children and young adults. They frequently have powerful side-effects which can include worsening of psychological states, suicide and aggressive outbursts. Their use should never be considered lightly and it is helpful to consider gentler options first. They are easy to begin but more difficult to stop. They are addictive and stopping them can lead to withdrawal symptoms as well as a flare-up of the original symptoms.

Many people feel that the personality produced by antidepressants is not a real or useful one. It also has the effect of making people who take it develop the same personality, *'shiny, happy people'* as Professor David Rothman has described them. He sees *'a danger of it being used as a method of pharmacologically induced social control'*. It would be more accurate to acknowledge that this is what is already happening.

The use of antidepressants is a direct result of conventional medicine's belief that depression is caused by physical abnormalities in the brain that can be corrected by the use of physical agents – drugs, electroshock and so forth. There is no evidence that this is the case.

The danger of an emphasis on physical matters is that psychological states may be given little attention. People are dismissed as being neurotic, invariably used as a pejorative term, and applied more readily to women than men. Drugs are frequently prescribed in an attempt to 'rebalance' supposed chemical abnormalities in the substance of the brain. There is a fostering of the misunderstanding that psychological difficulties can only be remedied by external forces, either a doctor or medication prescribed by a doctor. As psychiatrist Thomas Szasz once said, *'Trying to get rid of a so-called mental illness by having a psychiatrist work on your brain is like trying to get cigarette commercials off television by having a TV repairman work on your TV set.'*

If you are taking antidepressant medication, it will be most helpful to consult with a qualified practitioner for guidance. It is possible to reduce or stop medication in most cases with appropriate support and help although you should never stop medication suddenly. Clearly, it is more complex to deal with situations complicated by the use of prescribed drugs. If in doubt, seek help and advice.

PICTURES OF DEPRESSION

A man of 45 years develops symptoms of irritability and sleep disturbance, particularly waking in the night. This developed after a long period of working long hours in a stressful job. He sighs a lot, is impatient and suffers from a lowness of mood as well as feelings of low esteem.

A woman of 25 years has a miscarriage when she is 15 weeks pregnant. After feeling very happy at being pregnant, she feels very sad and low. She weeps easily and has feelings of tightness in the chest.

A woman of 55 years reports symptoms of tiredness, poor memory, lack of concentration and depressed feelings. She finds it difficult to think clearly and finds that she churns things over and over in her mind. She has a poor appetite.

A man of 60 years complains of depressed feelings with tiredness. He also complains of low back ache with some frequent urination. Everything he tries to do is an effort, indeed, he cannot see the point of doing anything.

All these people may be given a label of 'depression' despite their quite different symptoms. In conventional medicine, they may all be given the same or similar antidepressants. There may be a belief that such chemicals can treat a 'chemical imbalance' in the brain that leads to such symptoms. Whilst treatment with antidepressants may be appropriate in certain situations where symptoms are particularly severe, there is no evidence to suppose that depression arises from such a chemical imbalance .

In holistic medicine, we seek to give each person an individual remedy precisely tailored to their particular pattern of symptoms. I will discuss this in more detail later when recommending different remedies to help alleviate depression.

A DIFFERENT POINT OF VIEW

When dealing with any psychological symptom, including depression, there are two aspects of mind that it is helpful to consider.

There is the mind that is discursive, distracted and always getting ourselves (and others) into difficulty and dissatisfaction. At the same time, there is the Mind that can be likened to the sky on a cloudless day – the unchanging aspect of ourselves that is beyond all suffering and discomfort.

The usual thoughts and emotions of our everyday experience can be considered similar to the clouds that appear in the sky from time to time. They are not the sky itself but merely obscure it. They come and go. It is when we are attached to the clouds of our thoughts and emotions that we begin to experience suffering. If we can begin to realise that all events are merely a manifestation of constantly changing causes and conditions, then we become less worried and attached to the constantly changing environment of our minds. Nothing is static and permanent.

Treatment is particularly effective if people are encouraged to see their psychological processes for what they are – impermanent and constantly changing. They are not 'us', not our Mind, they are merely transitory. In this way, people become less attached to problems and suffering and can experience periods of comfort and ease. Approaches that directly deal with inner states are the most powerful methods of transformation. Visualisation and meditation are just some of the methods that can be used.

LIFESTYLE FACTORS

In the modern world, it is common to find that people overuse their mental functions. Long working hours, going to bed late, eating poor quality food, eating on the move or irregularly, all tend to be common. The energy becomes exhausted especially, in traditional Chinese medicine (TCM) terms, the energy of the digestion and kidneys. There is no time for us to rest and replenish our stores. Even at night in cities, constant noise is absorbed and our minds cannot rest during sleep. One of the most effective methods for strengthening ourselves mentally and emotionally is by meditation. Others include getting adequate rest, eating a healthy and nutritious diet, developing harmonious and supportive relationships and avoiding activities which deplete our energy.

RECOGNISING DEEP SEATED ISSUES

In the West, particularly, psychological disturbances can be deep-seated. They frequently arise out of infancy and childhood. We are often brought up in environments that may be emotionally deprived and conflict ridden. These environments expose us to inappropriate influences, often at an early age. A common 'inappropriate' influence is abuse. This may be sexual and is frequently emotional. 20 per cent of women who had been sexually abused as a child have mental health problems, as opposed to 6.3 per cent of the non-abused population. Almost half of psychiatric in-patients have histories of sexual/physical abuse.

Deep-seated issues are not going to be completely remedied by treatment with holistic medicine over some weeks or even months. Although we all have witnessed remarkable success stories where genuine transformations have taken place rapidly, for most people, the process is more gradual. The point is that by choosing to act, making some lifestyle changes such as introducing regular meditation, and choosing a natural remedy will start the process. This action is in itself empowering and in conjunction with the supportive effects of the appropriate natural remedy real benefits can begin to be experienced. There may be setbacks but for most people, once the lifestyle suggestions and remedies have had a chance to take effect, you will be able to look back on your experience and see that you are less depressed and that real progress has been made.

FINDING HELPFUL APPROACHES

Psychological approaches can be invaluable in giving people extra help, including counselling and psychotherapy. Care, however, has to be taken in selecting the right approach for you. My view is that this may be counterproductive if it is too cathartic, too confrontational, and too invasive. The mind is complex, its neuroses so rich and varied, we can dig forever and come up with a problem or difficulty to be analysed. This is not necessarily helpful. The important issue is how to encourage people to recognise their own wisdom and clarity. As the Tibetans say, *'If the dung is dry, do not stir it.'* Gentle methods of transformation are usually more helpful than constant identification with the problem: identification with the solution is more beneficial. It is, in any case, the approach of the therapist that is the key; *'it is not what you do but the way that you do it'*. There are some contact addresses at the end of this booklet.

WHAT YOU CAN DO

A major aspect of this booklet is to encourage people in using techniques that can relieve the symptoms of depression.

I discuss depression in different ways as it varies from person to person. In this way, you can relate your own situation or that of a loved one to the descriptions here. You can then determine an approach that may prove beneficial.

As a first strategy, consider:
- a simple meditation or relaxation practice
- therapeutic herbs, flower essences or other therapies
- exercise
- a healthy diet

Later think about refining your approach to consider the different types described under 'Specific Patterns of Depression'.

This booklet is not intended to teach you how to self-diagnose but merely to become aware of symptoms, learn how to understand them in more depth and to use holistic approaches. Bear in mind that people with depression may need help and support from several sources.

SENSIBLE USE

Self-help can be applied safely and effectively in many situations. This is certainly true of the methods described below, however, there are times when professional help is necessary. This booklet is not intended to teach you how to deal with very strong symptoms.

Seek professional help if:
- symptoms are severe
- symptoms come on rapidly and get worse quickly
- symptoms get progessively worse over a period of days, weeks or months
- other symptoms begin to develop
- symptoms do not respond to your strategy of self-help
- you have a history of mental illness
- hallucinations or delusions are suspected
- you experience suicidal thoughts or urges
- there is progressive weight loss and/or disappearance of periods in women

MEDITATION

This is extremely helpful as such practices strengthen our minds, calm the spirit and provide mental and emotional stability.

Of all the methods available to us to be healthy, this is probably the most important. In a Chinese Han dynasty text it is stated, *"It is most important to nourish the spirit, it is of secondary importance to nourish the body. The spirit should be pure and tranquil, the bones should be stable. This is the foundation of long life."*

The Tibetans agree and say, *"The mind is King"*. It is the essential, innermost aspect of ourselves as human beings yet perhaps the most difficult to access. However, it is at the level of the mind that true miracles can occur. Meditation leads to an increased level of emotional and mental well-being due to its ability to directly transform negative states of mind. If meditation is new to you, or you are not confident about what you are doing see page 24 for some suggestions of meditation techniques.

HERBS

Herbal medicine has a long and proven track record in alleviating suffering and maximising health.

'Over the counter' herbs are generally safe and gentle as well as effective and can be easily used for self-help. It is helpful to consult a qualified herbalist if you find that your strategy of self-help does not help or in more complicated cases where symptoms are severe. Anyone taking prescribed medication should also see a practitioner before using herbal remedies.

ST. JOHN'S WORT *(Hypericum perforatum)*

This herb is well known to relieve mild to moderate depression and in clinical trials has been proven to be more effective than placebo and better tolerated than antidepressants . It is also specifically indicated to relieve the 'winter blues' (SAD). It may be taken as an infusion, tincture or as capsules. There are certain prescribed drugs that interact with St. John's Wort: these include oral contraception, antidepressant medication, certain antibiotics and HIV medication. Check with a practitioner before using if you also take prescription drugs.

DAMIANA *(Turnera diffusa)*

Damiana is a stimulant and tonic to the nervous system and may be used to treat depression, physical weakness, difficulty thinking and nervous exhaustion. Damiana is also considered a stimulant for the reproductive system (aphrodisiac) in both sexes. It is best taken as an infusion or tincture.

LEMON BALM *(Melissa officinalis)*

This pleasant tasting herb is well-known as a lifter of mood, it treats the 'heart and driveth away melancholy and sadness' according to John Evelyn in the 17th century and new research into its antidepressant properties was presented to the British Psychological Society in April, 2004. Lemon balm lifts the spirits and also provides support for the nervous system during times of stress. Although effective, lemon balm is a mild herb that is suitable for children and adults. It is best taken as an infusion or tincture.

SKULLCAP *(Scutellaria lateriflora)*
Skullcap is a very effective herb that has a calming yet strengthening effect on the nervous system and will help to relieve certain symptoms of depression such as poor sleep, poor concentration and headaches. It is particularly useful for depression brought on by prolonged stress, illness or overwork. Skullcap may be taken as an infusion, capsules or tincture.

All the herbs above may be taken for up to six weeks at a time. It is usually advisable to then have a break for a couple of weeks before taking for another six weeks if required. The herbs may be taken in combination.

If you develop any new symptoms or are unsure about your progress consult a qualified herbalist who will be able to tailor an exact prescription to your needs and get a deeper result. During pregnancy or if you are on prescribed medication check with a practitioner before taking herbal remedies.

An infusion is made by adding a heaped teaspoonful of herb (or herbs) to a pot and pouring on a cupful of boiling water. Allow this to infuse for 10 minutes, strain and drink 3 times per day. A tincture is an extract of herb in alcohol and water. The usual dosage is 1 to 2ml in a glass of water 3 times per day, follow the dosage instructions on the bottle.

FLOWER ESSENCES

These are made from flowers and are very gentle in relieving negative states of mind. They are not addictive and do not interact with any other treatments or prescribed medication. I often recommend them to help with difficult emotions. The best-known ones are the Bach Flower Remedies and the following blends are all based on Bach Flower Remedies.

The following blends have been developed by Julian Barnard of the Flower Essence Program and can be mixed yourself by adding each of the individual remedies listed to a dropper bottle, or they can be purchased ready-mixed from Neal's Yard Remedies.

COURAGE

This blend encourages calm control and courage when fears and apprehensions have taken over. It gently dispels fearfulness and inner turmoil so feelings of security and safety can take root.

Indicated for: panic, fears, shyness, trembling, fear for others or the world, fear of hurting self or others, mental torment.

Contains: honeysuckle, cherry plum, mimulus, red chestnut, rock rose, aspen, agrimony.

CONFIDENCE & POWER

Supports assertiveness and inner strength when life's challenges have sapped motivation and esteem. It brings a stronger sense of individuality & the ability to function with more integrity.

Indicated for: poor sense of self, belittling, apologetic, lack of confidence, powerlessness, inferiority, submissive, discouraged, self-sacrificing.

Contains: larch, centaury, rock rose, gentian, elm, pine.

DIRECTION

A supporting blend during times of personal transformation when direction may be lost and it can be harder to make decisions. Promotes clarity and increased self understanding.

Indicated for: lack of commitment, mid-life crisis, career changes, doubt, indecision, apathy, fear of future, lack of responsibility.

Contains: scleranthus, wild oat, cerato, walnut, mimulus, wild rose.

FOCUS

Helps clear the head, increase confidence in the self and bring a positive attitude to learning and academic work. It can help focus the mind if under the pressure of deadlines.

Indicated for: exams. Interviews, cramming, mental tiredness, overwhelmed, fear of failure, revision, distracted, fuzzy-headed, mental chatter, uninspired.

Contains: larch, elm, white chestnut, hornbeam, gentian, clematis.

LETTING GO

Promotes acceptance and understanding when anger and bitterness seem uppermost in the mind and it's difficult to feel life is fair. Could also bring essential insight into the self.

Indicated for: resentment, intolerance, co-dependence, neediness, unhappiness, relationship problems, attention seeking, blaming, indifference, uncaring, distancing, controlling, won't change.

Contains: holly, willow, vine, beech, chicory, water violet.

OPTIMISM

Brings a renewal of optimism and faith when life feels impossible. It brings about a gentle rebirth as it uplifts the self out of intense darkness and into the light.

Indicated for: moodiness, gloom, despondence, adolescents, discouraged, hopelessness, pessimistic, despairing, dark-night of the soul, loneliness.

Contains: gorse, gentian, mustard, sweet chestnut, cherry plum, heather.

REVITALISE

Brings strength and energy when life's responsibilities have taken their toll and fatigue has set in. It helps a depleted system recuperate by making available essential support & vitality.

Indicated for: debilitated, burn-out, overworked, carers, strained, women's cycles, drained, no get up and go, overwhelmed, low, fragile, weak, out of sorts.

Contains: olive, elm, oak, crab apple, hornbeam, walnut.

UNWIND

Brings welcome relief when it becomes increasingly difficult to relax, switch off and recharge with a refreshing nights sleep.

Indicated for: stressed, uptight, overwrought, striving, impatience, perfectionism, worry, restless nights, working too hard.

Contains: vervain, impatiens, agrimony, rock water, walnut, aspen, white chestnut.

S.O.S

Dr Bach's classic rescue combination promotes feelings of calm and serenity and is for life's most extreme challenges or situations. Frequent use is suggested during those times.

Indicated for: emergencies, bereavement, interviews, life dramas, emotional situations, travel, public speaking, exam nerves, anguish.

Contains: clematis, impatiens, rock rose, star of Bethlehem, cherry plum.

AROMATHERAPY

Essential oils have a complex action on the body that is still not fully understood.

This may be due to the fact that one oil can have hundreds of different compounds. Interestingly, your sense of smell is over 10,000 more sensitive than your sense of taste and researchers have shown how aromas cause a brain reaction, activating the hypothalamus gland, the pituitary gland and the body's hormones as well as stimulating the limbic system (centre for emotion and memory) in the brain.

During a visit to an aromatherapist, they will first take a case history, understanding what particular symptoms you experience. A carefully selected blend of essential oils will then be blended for your aromatherapy massage. The aromatherapist is likely to choose from essential oils that are known to relieve symptoms of anxiety and tension, such as lavender and chamomile and those that have an uplifting antidepressant action such as neroli and rose.

There have been a number of clinical trials demonstrating the effectiveness of regular aromatherapy massage treatments in improving the symptoms of depression. In one particular trial in the UK in 2006, all the recorded symptoms of depression including low mood, anxiety and tension were significantly improved in those receiving aromatherapy massage once a week for six weeks compared to those receiving no massage.

HOMŒOPATHY

The correct homœopathic remedy acts like a key, unlocking a flow of insights and energy that has previously been held back.

Although physical complaints can be greatly relieved by homœopathic treatment, often the first improvements observed by the patient after treatment is that their energy improves, they feel a lift in spirits and generally 'better in themselves'.

Although you can purchase homœopathic remedies over the counter to treat yourself for minor ailments, choosing the right series of remedies for yourself for something complex like depression is not easy, and best results will come from visiting a practitioner. Most qualified homœopaths will have experience of successfully treating people with depression, and this is a therapy that has played an important role in overcoming depression for many people. To find a qualified homœopath near you see the list of contacts at the back of the book.

EXERCISE

Regular exercise has been proven conclusively to have a beneficial effect in relieving symptoms of anxiety and depression.

The physically active are less likely to suffer less from stress and depression than the non-active. Exercise is so effective at relieving symptoms of depression for a number of reasons: including increased release of endorphins (the hormones associated with feeling happy), reduced muscle and nervous tension, as well as the improvement of self-esteem, improved concentration, and, obviously, physical fitness.

The important thing is to get started and keep it going regularly, to get into a positive energy cycle rather than a negative loop. Obviously when you are feeling depressed it is difficult to feel motivated to take exercise but bear in mind the words of Dr Blumenthal, an American professor of medical psychology that, *"exercise seems to be at least as effective as standard antidepressant medications in reducing symptoms in patients with depression"*.

Walking, cycling, swimming, playing sport at a low level, gardening and line dancing have all been shown to be effective forms of exercise for relieving symptoms: it is a moderate level of exercise that is required. Moderate exercise will mean you may become slightly breathless, and you will need to exercise for about 30 minutes a day, 5-6 days a week.

DIET

It seems that there are more diet books than people these days and we could follow a different diet for every day of the month.

Is there any wonder that we can become confused about what to eat, when to eat, how to eat or whether to eat at all? I do not intend to give you yet another complicated list of advice as to eating which will then be forgotten by the time you have put this booklet down.

Remember that food is about enjoyment. If we do not enjoy what we eat, then it is hardly likely to give us health and nourish us. We may have very fixed ideas as to what is healthy and what is not. There are very few foods that are inherently unhealthy: a more important question is, 'What is healthy for me'? We are all individuals and we vary from person to person as to what is healthy. The key is moderation. If we eat well for most of the time, that is fine.

The essence of a healthy diet is to eat fresh food regularly. In a cool temperate climate such as Northern Europe, it is better to eat mainly warm food, especially during the winter. This is to protect the energy of the digestion which is already working hard to keep us warm. It is helpful to think about using culinary herbs that are warming and energizing, such as rosemary, thyme and ginger. Salads are fine in the warmer weather, and if you live in a hot climate.

Eat regularly three times daily. The old adage, *'Breakfast like a king, lunch like a prince and supper like a pauper'* fits in better with our activity and the energy of our digestion which is strongest between 7 and 11 in the morning.

Some other helpful guidelines include:
- Eat fresh food.
- Eat mainly warm food especially in the winter. Fresh root ginger and garlic add extra warmth to a dish.
- Porridge is ideal for breakfast – oat, millet or rice.
- Eat lots of soups and casseroles.
- Eat plenty of fresh fruit and vegetables. You can bake or stew fruit with ginger and/or cinnamon.

- Eat as much organically grown food as possible, this will have less synthetic contaminants present and a higher mineral content from healthier soil.

A certain amount of meat can be considered beneficial to eat although white meat (fish or chicken) is generally easier to digest. As a nation we generally eat more meat protein than is necessary for health so try reducing meat to every second day and use other sources of protein on other days.

Foods to avoid completely or to greatly reduce are sugar, coffee, alcohol, refined or processed foods, fizzy drinks, bleached white grains such as white bread, white pasta.

Essential Fatty Acids

Studies have reported that countries with high rates of fish oil consumption have low rates of depressive disorder (Werbach, 1999). High consumption of unhealthy saturated fats (usually from fried food and animal fats) is thought to increase the incidence of depressive states, as is an imbalance in the intake of omega-6 and omega-3 essential fatty acids (EFA's). This imbalance is associated with a relatively higher consumption of omega-6 and lower consumption of omega-3 EFA's.

Hemp seed oil is a natural food source that contains the desired ratio of omega-3 and omega-6 EFA's, and can be used over the long tem to maintain a healthy EFA balance. Buy cold-pressed organic hemp seed oil and add to smoothies, soups and salad dressings.

Good sources of omega-3 EFA include cold water oily fish (such as salmon, mackerel and sardines). To correct an omega-3 essential fatty acid deficiency eat a variety of oily fish three times per week, or supplement with a good quality fish oil supplement.

Alternatively, a good vegetarian / vegan source of omega-3 essential fatty acids are linseeds (also called flax seeds). Crush and sprinkle one tablespoon of linseeds onto your breakfast of muesli, cereal or porridge every day or take 1 tablespoon of the cold pressed oil daily.

Other nutritional considerations include blood sugar imbalance, lack of chromium, lack of amino acids and lack of B vitamins. A nutrition consultant can help identify any factors that can be corrected by nutrition.

RESTORING BALANCE

Health has been described as our greatest gift. Each of us wants to know how to keep ourselves in the best state of health and well-being – both physically and psychologically.

Holistic medicine has a unique view of the whole person as an interconnecting energetic network. There are many different techniques that are encompassed within the term holistic medicine, and they are increasingly being recognised as great resources for promoting health and treating disease.

Holistic medicine has never sought to separate body and mind. These are seen as being inextricably linked and in recent times we have begun to rediscover this in the West.

Consequently, in holistic medicine, we have a positive view of health and being human. Health is not just the absence of symptoms but the presence of a vital and dynamic state of well-being. You may know from your own experience that there are times when you feel 'under the weather' or below par. You do not have a disease and but there is something not quite right. Holistic medicine is able to explain such feelings and has methods that can correct them.

ENERGY SYSTEMS

The key point about holistic medicine is that it is based upon the principle that there is an energy that flows through us and beyond us.

It has different names according to the particular form of holistic medicine that is being practised. It is the *Qi* of Chinese medicine, *Ki* in Japanese medicine, *prana* in Ayurvedic medicine, vital force in homœopathy and so forth.

Such energy flows through the body giving life to all tissues and organs along its path. It is considered that one's health is dependent on three factors, the smooth flow of energy, a good quality of energy and the correct functioning of the organs.

In terms of psychological health, the major organs of the body each have a different role in thoughts and emotions, in their healthy functioning and the maintenance of balance. For example, the Kidneys are related to the emotion of fear and to the will or ambition. If the Kidneys are imbalanced or weakened for whatever reason, we may experience phobias, general feelings of fear or perhaps an unbalanced sense of ambition. This can manifest either as 'driven' activity in order to achieve success – the typical workaholic – or as a depression or apathy where we cannot feel enthusiastic about ourselves or our surroundings.

In terms of traditional Chinese medicine, each of the five major organs, Liver, Heart, Kidney, Spleen and Lung have aspects that correspond to the mind and emotions as well as their physical function.

Organ	Mental aspect	Emotional aspect
Liver	Kindly & giving attitude, sharing	Anger, jealousy, guilt, assertiveness, resentment
Heart	Responsibility, gratitude, appreciation, politeness, humility	Joy, happiness
Kidney	Intellect, intelligence, wisdom, insight, will power, ambition	Fear
Spleen	Belief, faith, confidence, trust	Sympathy
Lung	Sensibility, compassion, attitude, sensitiveness, vulnerability	Grief, sadness

It can be seen that emotions such as depression may arise from several sources. It may be sadness and grief due to a Lung imbalance or a lack of joy from the Heart. It may be apathy due to lack of ambition relating to the Kidney. There may be a simmering anger or resentment due to a Liver imbalance or a churning, rumination from the Spleen. It is essential, therefore, whatever the prime, presenting symptom, that everybody is treated as an individual.

SPECIFIC PATTERNS OF DEPRESSION

The precise nature of our symptoms depends upon the particular organ that is affected.

I have listed a simple classification below, based on traditional Chinese medicine, that indicates different types of depression and suggested the holistic approach that will best help.

TYPE 1 – THE LUNG TYPE

In Chinese medicine the Lung is associated with letting go. Symptoms are depression that is characterised by sadness, sometimes accompanied with anxiety, weeping and sighing. There may be a history of loss such as a bereavement. There may be other symptoms of pale face, tiredness, cough, tightness in the chest and, in severe cases, breathlessness.

Diet: a generally healthy diet as described above with the addition of steamed foods to benefit the Lung. Also, eat soups, chicken, dates, honey, malt.

Breathing is very important in this situation to open the chest and remove any energetic blockages to breathing. Yoga, tai chi or qi gong are all of great benefit and also the breathing relaxation practice as described above.

Herbs: consider codonopsis root, ginseng and astragalus, which are all available as tinctures or may be boiled up and taken as a drink or soup.

TYPE 2 – THE LIVER TYPE

There may be a general feeling of not being able to move forward in your life. There is a 'stuckness'. The Liver is associated with the smooth flow of *Qi*. There will be associated symptoms of anger, irritability, lack of patience, frustration and resentment. In women, there may be pre-menstrual symptoms of headaches, sore and distended breasts and painful periods. Headaches at the side of the head, belching, sighing, indigestion and difficulty getting off to sleep at night are often seen in Liver-type depressions.

Diet: a generally healthy diet as described above with the addition of foods such as basil, caraway, cardamon, carrot, cayenne, chive, clove, coriander, dill seed, garlic, marjoram, orange and tangerine peel, radish, turmeric. Going on a cleansing or detox diet for a period of time may help. Take hot lemon each morning

– squeeze the juice of a quarter of a lemon into a mug with hot water and a teaspoon of honey, drink when warm.

TYPE 3 – THE SPLEEN TYPE

The thoughts and emotions may be overactive and merely 'churn over'. They occupy our mind but do not actually go anywhere. This is to do with the Spleen which deals with transformation, not just food but also mental and emotional states.

Depression arising from this organ is to do with a not moving, an inability to 'digest' thoughts and emotions. There may be associated symptoms of poor appetite, loose stools, nausea and tiredness.

Diet: a generally healthy diet as described above with no cold, or raw food. Eat foods which are warm in energy such as basil, beef, chestnuts, chicken, clove, coconut, dates, dill, fennel seed, garlic, ginger, grapes, ham, kidney, lamb, lentil, mackerel, molasses, mushroom (shiitake), nutmeg, oats, potato, rabbit, raspberry, rosemary, sage, soybean curd (tofu), squash, sweet potato, thyme, walnut, yam.

Herbs: use codonopsis, ginseng, astragalus as tinctures or boiled up as a drink or soup.

TYPE 4 – THE HEART TYPE

There may be a feeling of unhappiness and a sense of loneliness. There is a general lack of *joie de vivre*. Associated symptoms include palpitations, insomnia, anxiety and discomfort in the chest. Severe cases may be associated with strong feelings of unworthiness and even suicidal thoughts.

Diet: a generally healthy diet as described above with the addition of foods such as apple, apricot, asparagus, beans (aduki, green, kidney), beef, beetroot, cheese, dandelion, dates, duck, egg, grapes, honey, leaf greens, liver, malt, mango, milk, nettle, parsley, pea, pear, pineapple, pork, spinach, sweet rice, soybean curd (tofu), tomato, watercress, watermelon, yam.

Herbs: angelica, fleeceflower root as tinctures or boiled up as a drink or soup.

TYPE 5 – THE KIDNEY TYPE

Depression may be more a case of lack of drive and ambition. There is an apathy, a lack of direction in our lives and a feeling of 'can't be bothered'. Phobias or more generalised fear of things may be present. In severe cases there may deep despair. This can alternate with periods of excessive drive and overwork. The Kidneys are associated with the Will and ambition depends upon this organ.

Diet: a generally healthy diet as described above with the addition of walnuts and chestnuts plus if you are not a vegetarian a small amount of sliced lamb's kidney in a soup or with rice once a week.

Do not stand or sit for long periods, try to move around every 30 minutes or so. Avoid heavy lifting and keep your lower back warm at all times.

SUMMARY

- Psychological disorders are extremely common.
- People with depression may need help and support from several sources.
- Counselling and psychotherapy, of an appropriate nature, can be extremely beneficial in helping people resolve psychological issues.
- It is helpful if our thoughts and emotions can be viewed within the whole perspective of human experience and its possibilities, not just to see them as something 'negative' and to be 'got rid of'.

APPENDICES

MEDITATION TECHNIQUES

What is meditation? Simply, it is a state of mind that does not seek to manipulate thoughts and emotions but merely to allow them to settle of their own accord.

For some people, this may occur as they are absorbed in some simple task or when they are in a particularly relaxed state of mind. If this is the case with yourself, use that feeling when you begin the meditation exercises described below.

As the thoughts and emotions settle, the natural clarity of the mind is revealed and its natural radiance, which is compassion, will shine out.

What then is mind? There are many levels of mind or consciousness. There are two to consider here. The ordinary or judgmental mind is frequently the mind of our everyday existence and the one that leads us into all sorts of difficulties and problems. It seeks to see the world in terms of dualities, of good and bad, of achievement and failure, etc. It is this mind that reacts to situations with anger, irritation, impatience, jealousy and so forth.

The innermost level of mind has different terms according to the particular spiritual or religious tradition – God, Buddha nature, the Tao, Allah, are all terms which essentially mean the same thing, that innermost aspect of ourselves which is beyond suffering. This mind can be considered to be sky-like in nature, yet aware, clear, unobstructed and limitless in its wisdom and compassion.

IS IT HARD?

Meditation can be learnt and practiced by anyone because we all have a mind. The methods I describe here are simple ways for anyone of whatever spiritual or religious inclination to allow the mind to calm and to settle.

When you first begin to meditate you may notice that your mind becomes noisier and busier. This shows that the meditation is working because you have started to become aware of the 'internal chatter' that is not normally noticed in our busy lives. With time, thoughts settle and emotions are calmed.

MEDITATION POSTURE

The most important thing about the posture is that the back should be upright so that the spine is vertical. The back is traditionally said to be like a 'pile of golden coins' or 'straight as an arrow'.

The head is slightly inclined downwards and the gaze softly focused in front. The tradition of meditation I am familiar with teaches that the eyes should be open. This is so that we are not cut off from the world but can integrate all of our experiences. If you find it more comfortable to begin with the eyes closed then do so although this may lead to sleepiness. If tiredness is a problem just open the eyes slightly to increase your alertness. If your mind becomes overactive, you may find it helpful to lower your gaze.

Sit on an upright chair or cross-legged on the floor. The important thing is to be comfortable. 'Lotus' positions for the legs are not necessary at the beginning of practice.

Relax the body and breathing and release any areas of tension particularly in the neck, jaw and shoulders. The tip of the tongue touches the roof of the mouth behind the upper teeth. This is to connect the energy flow round the body. Breathe softly and gently through the mouth and nose.

EXERCISE ONE - BREATHING RELAXATION

This exercise is a simple method of breathing in a relaxed manner and using the whole of the lungs. It is known as abdominal or diaphragmatic breathing and is associated with relaxation.

When we are tense, we breathe using our upper chest. Bringing the breath down into the abdomen makes our breathing more efficient and releases deeply held tensions.

Either use the meditation posture above or lie down in a comfortable and warm place. Gently close your eyes or have them slightly open and softly focused a short distance in front of you.

As you breathe in, let your abdomen expand and your chest remain still. In this way, the diaphragm moves down, the lungs expand and air is drawn into them.

As you breathe out, let your abdomen move in so that air is expelled from your lungs.

You may find it helpful to have a hand on your upper chest and abdomen. This is useful as you begin, to help you keep the chest stable and for breathing to take place in the abdomen. Later on, as it becomes more natural you will find you can merely have your hands relaxed in your lap or resting by your side.

FOCUS OF MEDITATION

There are several things that you can use as a focus during your meditation. Two that I want to discuss here are the breath and an object.

EXERCISE TWO - FOCUSING ON THE BREATH

Read the section above dealing with the posture of meditation. Then try this exercise which will gently focus on the breath.

As you breathe in and out, gently become aware of the flow of breath entering and leaving your body.

As you breathe out, release any tension or feelings of discomfort that you experience.

As you breathe in, allow the breath to soften and release any areas of tension or discomfort. With each in-breath and out-breath you become more and more relaxed.

As thoughts and emotions arise in the mind, do not follow them, do not become involved in them, merely watch them rise and fall.

EXERCISE THREE - FOCUSING ON AN OBJECT

This is very similar to the meditation above. You can use any object for your focus although try to find something which you find inspiring. This could be a flower, a beautiful picture, a religious figure, a candle flame, a photograph or painting from nature, whatever connects with you.

As you calm your mind, gently focus on the object. Allow your mind to settle and peacefully relax. Whenever you find that you are distracted, gently bring your attention back to the object.

EXERCISE FOUR - VISUALISATION

Visualisation is using the mind to imagine a situation that will then come into being. If we want to learn a certain occupation, we imagine or visualise what it would be like to do that work and be that person. This is the crucial first stage. Similarly, with regards to our health, we can visualise our bodies as being healthy and whole.

Use the meditation posture described above. The straight spine ensures that *Qi* and Blood flow as harmoniously as possible. Relax your body and mind. Pay attention to any areas of tension in your body. Check over each area of your body in turn. Common areas which collect tension are the jaw, neck and shoulders and the chest area.

As you breathe in, imagine breathing in white light. This is healing and cooling and energising. Each time you breathe in, you breathe in more and more healing light. Particularly concentrate on areas of tension or discomfort. If you have a specific disease, you can pay particular attention to sending healing light to that area.

As you breathe out, visualise all tension, discomfort and problems leaving your body as dark smoke. Each breath causes more dark smoke to leave you.

So, with each in-breath, you take in healing light which dissolves tension, discomfort and disease. With each out-breath, you breathe out dark smoke and so removing tension, discomfort and disease.

Continue this practice for as long as you can until your whole body has been filled by white light and totally healed. All problems have been removed and your body is now shining with white healing and energising light.

Two suggestions for more effective practice:
- Make sure that when you finish the practice, you have a sense that all problems have been removed. Do not leave a little bit over until the next time.
- Practice daily for maximum benefit.

MEDITATION IN YOUR DAILY LIFE

All the teachers and meditation masters agree that it is regular practice which produces the greatest results. With meditation and visualisation for a specific health problem, the degree of recovery is directly related to the amount of time spent in meditation. Regular practice is the key and meditating daily will have definite, measurable results.

However, when we begin to practice, it can be immensely difficult to find the time. We lead busy lives with many distractions and meditation can be the last thing we come to even though we may know of its benefits.

Practice meditation for an amount of time each day which is comfortable for you. There is no set time which you have to practice for. To begin with, perhaps 5 or 10 minutes is enough. It is better to start with a small amount which is manageable than to fail at a longer time. The time of day when you practice should be to suit you. You may find that practising in the morning is more helpful because our energy is fresher and stronger then, although you may have more time in the evening.

Consider the environment of your meditation. Choose a favourite place in your house or in the garden. Meditating in the outdoors in direct contact with nature can be very inspiring and greatly benefit our practice. Perhaps have a small area in your house or bedroom which is devoted to meditation. Consider using flowers, a beautiful picture, lighting incense or having an inspiring object in your meditation area which can help you. Meditation provides an inspiring environment for your mind. It can be helped by providing such an environment in your physical surroundings.

The main point here is that you are creating a space for your meditation to occur and this is reflected in a space within your mind. Thus, thoughts and emotions settle allowing your inner clarity to arise.

FINDING A MEDITATION TEACHER

The meditation exercises in this booklet can be applied easily and simply. With practice you will notice definite changes. You may reach a stage where you need further guidance or help in understanding your experiences in meditation. When you find a teacher, make an assessment of the person's qualifications and training. Discuss with them their particular tradition of meditation and where it comes from. Only accept guidance when you are satisfied that this person can give you what you need.

Many people find that meditation as part of a group brings them many benefits. This is something you can consider and discuss when looking into possible teachers. Taking part in a group meditation allows you to guage how suitable it is for you and perhaps learn about the experience of others with the practice.

HOW TO CHOOSE A PRACTITIONER

It is an important decision to seek help from a health practitioner and this is particularly so if the method of treatment is not one with which you are familiar.

It is generally emphasised to seek help from a registered practitioner. However, different countries have different regulations concerning this and some practitioners choose, for a variety of reasons not to be registered. They may be experienced and professional people so you need some system to check on individual practitioners.

It is essential that you consider their training. Where did the person train and how long was the training? There are a bewildering array of qualifications and certificates. Checking directly with the person is the best way to find out what they mean. Do not be afraid of asking people about this as your health is too important to leave in the hands of poorly qualified people.

INVOLVE YOURSELF IN TREATMENT

I would encourage you to be actively involved in your health program and discuss this with your practitioner. Ask questions but also take their recommendations. In this way, you will reap the benefits of the treatment more fully and quickly.

It would also be helpful to discuss at this time:
- the cost of treatment
- any extra charges for items such as herbs
- the probable duration of treatment
- how many appointments you can expect to need
- when and how to contact the practitioner

ATMOSPHERE OF TREATMENT

Treatment is not just about formal qualification and training. It is also about how you feel with this particular person. Healing takes place in an atmosphere of relaxation and with feelings of trust and security. This means that it is your personal connection with the practitioner (and theirs with you) which is the single most important thing to consider. You may be discussing quite personal feelings and thoughts and you are certainly experiencing a treatment which can affect people quite deeply. It is more effective and certainly more curative when you feel comfortable with the practitioner.

COST

The price of a treatment is dependent on many factors including location and the experience of the practitioner. Price is certainly something to check out before the consultation. Discuss it with your practitioner before attending so that you are clear about how much treatment will cost. It is usual to make additional charges for herbs.

SUMMARY

The important issues are:
- check on the training of a particular practitioner
- try to see someone who is personally recommended by a friend or another practitioner who you know
- discuss your case (including fees) with the practitioner before finally deciding upon treatment

FURTHER READING

The Healing Power of Illness by Dethlefsen, T. and D, Rudiger (Element, 1990)

Optimum Nutrition for the Mind by Patrick Holford (Piatkus, 2003)

Full Catastrophe Living by Jon Kabat-Zinn (Piatkus, 1996)

Families and How to Survive Them by Skynner and Cleese (Mandarin, 1990)

Law, Liberty, and Psychiatry by Thomas S. Szasz, M.D. (Syracuse Univ. Press, 1989)

Medical Nemesis by Ivan Illich (Penguin, 1995)

Psychiatric Drugs: Hazards to the Brain by Peter R. Breggin, M.D. (Springer Pub. Co. , 1983)

Your Drug May Be Your Problem: How and Why to Stop Taking Psychiatric Drugs by Breggin and Cohen (Perseus Books, 1999)

The Tibetan Book of Living and Dying by Sogyal Rinpoche (Rider, 2002)

Big Pharma: How the World's Biggest Drug Companies Control Illness by Jackie Law (Constable, 2006)

Beyond Prozac by Terry Lynch (Mercier, 2005)

Recipes for Self-Healing by Daverick Leggatt (Meridian Press, 1999)

SUPPLIERS

NEAL'S YARD REMEDIES
For your nearest shop contact 01747 834634 or www.
Mail order: 0845 262 3145
www.nealsyardremedies.com

Herbs, supplements, flower remedies, homœopathic remedies, information and practitioners.

HELIOS HOMŒOPATHY
89-97 Camden Road,
Tunbridge Wells, Kent
TN1 2QR
www.helios.co.uk
Tel: 01892 537254

Homœopathic remedies, flower remedies, information and practitioners.

AINSWORTH'S HOMŒOPATHIC PHARMACY
36 New Cavendish Street,
London
W1G 8UF
Tel: 020 7935 5330
www.ainsworths.com

CONTACTS

National Institute of Medical Herbalists
Elm House, 54 Mary Arches St,
Exeter, EX4 3BA
www.nimh.org.uk
Tel: 01392 426022

Dr Bach Flower Remedies
Healing Herbs Ltd
PO Box 65, Hereford
HR2 0DX
www.healingherbs.co.uk
Tel: 01873 890218

Register of Chinese Herbal Medicine
Office 5, 1 Exeter Street,
Norwich, NR2 4QB
www.rchm.co.uk
Tel: 01603 623994

British Acupuncture Council
63 Jeddo Road,
London, W12 9HQ
www.acupuncture.org.uk
Tel: 020 8735 0400

Society of Homeopaths
11 Brookfield, Duncan Close,
Moulton Park, Northampton,
NN3 6WL
www.homeopathy-soh.org
Tel: 0845 450 6611

Tai Chi and Qi Gong
Tse Qigong Centre
PO Box 59, Altrincham,
WA15 8FS
www.qimagazine.com
Tel: 0161 929 4485.

British Wheel of Yoga
25 Jermyn Street, Sleaford,
Lincolnshire,
NG34 7RU.
www.bwy.org.uk
Tel: 01529 306851

Mind (National Association for Mental Health)
15-19 Broadway, London
E15 4BQ
www.mind.org.uk
Tel: 020 8519 2122

Relate
Herbert Gray College,
Little Church Street, Rugby,
Warwickshire,
CV21 3AP.
www.relate.org.uk
Tel: 0845 456 1310 or
          01788 573241

Samaritans
www.samaritans.org
Tel: 08457 909090